ANDREA ABELLA MARIE

Understanding the Levels of Autism

A Quick Guide To The Challenges Each Level Faces, Strategies And Techniques That Can Assist Each Level, And Potential Resources For Those Levels

This book was professionally typeset on Reedsy.
Find out more at reedsy.com

"Autism is not a disability, it is a different ability."

Stuart Duncan

Contents

Acknowledgments

I would not be where I am today without the CEO of the company I work for. She gave me the opportunity to work in this field. That opportunity gave me the practical knowledge and skills I needed to succeed in this career path. She saw a need in the community and I was able to play a very small part in bridging the gap of that need. I am forever grateful to her.

I would like to thank my sister for helping me edit this book. I would also like to thank Rasmus and Christian Mikkelsen from Publishing.com who gave me the tools, resources, motivation, confidence, and drive that I needed to make this book happen. This book would not have been possible without them!

Introduction

Autism Spectrum Disorder (ASD) is a complex and multifaceted neurode-velopmental condition that affects millions of individuals worldwide. It is characterized by challenges in social communication, repetitive behaviors, and restricted interests, but it also encompasses a broad range of strengths and abilities. (American Psychiatric Association, 2013). Autism is not a one-size-fits-all diagnosis. Instead, it manifests uniquely in each individual, with varying degrees of severity and impacts on daily functioning. This diversity is why autism is referred to as a "spectrum" disorder.

Autism Spectrum Disorder (ASD) is one of the most varied developmental conditions, affecting individuals in unique and profound ways. While many people are familiar with the term "autism," fewer understand the breadth of the spectrum, or the varying levels of support required by those living with it. Autism affects communication, behavior, and social interaction. Its manifestation can range from subtle differences in social functioning to severe impairments requiring around-the-clock care.

Understanding autism requires not only knowledge of its characteristics but also empathy for the challenges these individuals face and a com-mitment to implementing effective strategies for support. That means acknowledging the unique challenges faced by those on the spectrum while exploring strategies to overcome these challenges that are specific to the individual and their needs. Understanding autism requires recognizing its nuances, including the different levels of support that individuals may require. By fostering a deeper understanding of autism, we can work towards creating an inclusive and supportive society where individuals with autism can thrive.

There is so much to the autism spectrum disorder (ASD). It is not possible to cover all the material in this short book. The goal of this book is to give a general overview of the three levels of the Autism Spectrum Disorder (ASD) while exploring the challenges faced by individuals at each level, and provide practical actionable strategies to overcome those challenges. Whether you are a caregiver, educator, healthcare professional, or simply someone seeking to learn more about autism, this book aims to equip you with some basic knowledge and a few actionable insights.

1

Chapter 1: What is Autism Spectrum Disorder (ASD)?

Defining ASD

Autism Spectrum Disorder (ASD) is a developmental condition that affects how individuals perceive and interact with the world. It is a lifelong condition that typically appears in early childhood, although it may not be diagnosed until later in life.

Autism Spectrum Disorder (ASD) is a condition characterized by persistent difficulties in social communication and restricted, repetitive patterns of behavior, interests, or activities. It is called a "spectrum" disorder because it encompasses a wide range of abilities, challenges, and support needs.

ASD can manifest in different ways. Some individuals may have significant challenges in communication and behavior, while others may experience subtle social difficulties that are less apparent. Autism is typically diagnosed in early childhood, but symptoms can be identified across the lifespan. Early intervention is key to improving outcomes. Understanding the different levels of ASD can help tailor support to each individual's needs.

ASD affects individuals in three primary areas:

1. **Social Communication** – It is shown by having difficulty in understanding and using verbal as well as nonverbal communication, leading to difficulties in social interactions. For instance, not being able to respond to a person who asks you a question.
2. **Repetitive Behaviors and Restricted Interests** – Demonstrated by patterns of repetitive actions and an intense focus on specific topics or activities. An example would be repeatedly opening and closing a backpacks zipper and only wanting to watch specific tv shows like SpongeBob.
3. **Sensory Processing** – Having atypical responses to sensory stimuli, such as a heightened sensitivity to noise and texture. This may manifest as aversions to foods and food restriction. Sometimes, individuals with this limitation can be seen covering their ears or turning the lights off.

Key Features of Autism

- **Social Communication Challenges:** Individuals with autism may struggle to interpret body language, gestures, facial expressions, and tone of voice. This can make it difficult to form relationships and participate in social activities.
- **Restricted Interests:** They may have a strong focus on specific topics or activities and exclude other activities or potential interests. Points of interest can range from hobbies, such as collecting or puzzles, to more abstract topics like maps or numbers.
- **Repetitive Behaviors:** Shown by engaging in repeated actions such as hand-flapping, lining up objects, rocking, or strict adherence to

routines. These behaviors are often comforting to individuals with ASD and can help them cope with stress or anxiety. These behaviors can also interfere with daily life.

- **Sensory Sensitivities:** Many individuals with autism have heightened or diminished responses to sensory input, such as sounds, lights, textures, or smells. This means an over- or under-responsiveness to things we take in with our senses, such as sound (ears), light (eyes), smell (nose), texture (taste), or temperature (touch). A heightened response can lead to sensory overload or avoidance. Sensory processing difficulties can make everyday environments overwhelming and challenging to navigate.

The Importance of Understanding the Spectrum

Autism is not a "one-size-fits-all" condition. No two individuals with autism are alike. This is why autism is categorized as a spectrum. Each individual with the disorder has unique strengths and challenges which makes it essential to tailor interventions to the individuals specific needs. Some may have profound challenges that require significant support, while others may excel academically or professionally despite subtle social difficulties. This diversity is another reason as to why it is referred to as a "spectrum disorder". Recognizing these differences is crucial to providing meaningful support because it allows for interventions that are both effective and respectful of an individual's autonomy and their personal goals.

2

Chapter 2: Levels of Autism

Overview of the DSM-5 Classification
The Diagnostic and Statistical Manual of Mental Disorders, Fifth Edition (DSM-5), categorizes autism into three levels based on the level of support required. The levels are:

1. **Level 1:** Requiring Support
2. **Level 2:** Requiring Substantial Support
3. **Level 3:** Requiring Very Substantial Support

These levels help clinicians determine the intensity of intervention required. The variance also assists caregivers in understanding what kind of support their loved ones may need. Thus, these levels help clinicians, caregivers, and educators better understand the specific needs of individuals and tailor interventions accordingly.

Note: You may find that there is some overlap between the different levels, particularly with levels 2 and 3. This is normal. Some information may seem repetitive but keep in mind that each level is different. Each level has varying degrees of severity with unique challenges and strategies of dealing with said challenges. It is also possible to use the same strategies, in varying degrees of capacity, with levels 2 and 3.

Characteristics of Each Level

Level 1 (Requiring Support):

Individuals at Level 1 may have mild social and communication difficulties. They may appear "high functioning" but still struggle with subtle aspects of social interaction. They may also have trouble adapting to changes in routine or behavior called behavioral rigidity. People at this level often have difficulty initiating and sustaining conversations, maintaining social relationships, interpreting social cues, and managing time effectively. Individuals at this level can typically carry employment and attend school but may require accommodations.

Level 2 (Requiring Substantial Support):

Individuals at Level 2 exhibit more pronounced difficulties in social communication and behavioral rigidity. Generally, they will have limited verbal and nonverbal communication skills. They often need substantial support to engage in activities of daily living because the behavioral rigidity and repetitive behaviors interfere with daily functioning. Individuals at this level may use limited language for communication and have difficulty coping with changes. They may benefit from structured environments and consistent routines such as following a daily schedule or plan. These individuals require consistent, structured support in most aspects of daily living. This is described as needing prompts in order to complete tasks. Prompts come in various degrees and forms. They may be verbal, gestural, visual, or physical. Employment at this level is possible with a job coach and short shifts such as 3 hours with a break in the middle.

Level 3 (Requiring Very Substantial Support):

This level is characterized by severe impairments in communication, behavior, and adaptability. Individuals often need constant support and care. People at Level 3 may be nonverbal or have minimal verbal abilities, requiring them to rely heavily on alternative communication methods. Their restricted interests and repetitive behaviors significantly impact their ability to engage in day-to-day activities. They typically require extensive assistance to complete daily tasks making it necessary to have around-the-clock care and support. For instance, they may need someone to help them use the bathroom, brush their teeth, get dressed, walk, and eat. This is described as needing physical prompting. Individuals at this level tend to thrive in predictable, highly structured settings. Generally, employment at this level is not possible. However, short volunteer opportunities with behavior technician's and BCBA's present can happen.

Why Levels Matter

Understanding the levels of autism helps caregivers, educators, and healthcare professionals develop tailored intervention plans that address each individual's unique challenges. The DSM-5 levels provide a framework that clarifies the amount of support needed in different aspects of life, whether it be in education, at home, or in social contexts. It also helps inform family members and others in the community about the most appropriate way to support individuals with autism.

3

Chapter 3: Challenges Faced by Individuals with Autism

There are many challenges faced by those diagnosed with Autism Spectrum Disorder. This chapter will go over some of the most common ones.

1. Communication Challenges

Communication barriers are one of the hallmark features of autism. The extent and nature of these barriers vary significantly from person to person.

- **Level 1:** Individuals may struggle with interpreting nonverbal cues, such as facial expressions and gestures. They may find it difficult to initiate conversations. Misunderstandings may arise due to their literal interpretation of language. They may monopolize conversations with their own special interests. Sarcasm, idioms, metaphors, and abstract language can be particularly confusing for individuals at Level 1.
- **Level 2:** Individuals at this level may have limited vocabulary and rely on repetitive phrases or scripted language. A lack of functional

language makes it harder to express even basic needs. They often struggle with reciprocal conversation. This means that they find it hard to keep conversations going and/or responding appropriately to others. Initiating communication can be a significant hurdle. Their difficulty in expressing emotions effectively can also impact their relationships.

- **Level 3:** Individuals at Level 3 often have minimal or no functional communication skills. They may be nonverbal or communicate primarily through gestures, body language, or augmentative alternative communication (AAC) devices. The inability to effectively communicate their needs and desires can lead to frustration and behavioral challenges.

2. Social Interaction Difficulties

Social difficulties are pervasive in individuals with autism, often leading to challenges in forming and maintaining relationships such as friendships. Social difficulties can lead to isolation and feelings of loneliness.

- **Level 1:** Individuals at this level may want to develop friendships but struggle with understanding societal norms and dynamics such as sharing interests or taking conversational turns. They may not know how to appropriately join into conversations or games, leading to feelings of rejection, social isolation, or rigidly rehearsed interactions. Anxiety in social situations is common, which can further hinder interactions.
- **Level 2:** Individuals at this level often display limited interest in social interactions. They have difficulty initiating conversations. They may interact primarily for practical reasons (e.g., to ask for help) rather than to connect emotionally with others. Understanding unspoken rules of social engagement is particularly challenging, and

they often need explicit instructions to navigate social situations.

- **Level 3:** Individuals at Level 3 usually show minimal engagement with others, even caregivers. They may even prefer solitary activities or interacting only with caregivers. Social interactions can be overwhelming for them. This may lead to distress and/or meltdowns, especially if they involve unfamiliar people or settings. Building meaningful relationships is often highly challenging without intensive support.

3. Behavioral Challenges

Repetitive behaviors and rigidity are common in autism and can significantly affect daily functioning.

- **Level 1:** Individuals may exhibit rigidity in thinking and behavior. They often have trouble shifting their focus from one task to another. They may become fixated on specific interests. They may also resist changes to their routines, which can lead to anxiety and frustration. Emotional regulation may be difficult as well. Even minor frustrations may trigger meltdowns.
- **Level 2:** Individuals at this level often display frequent meltdowns when routines are disrupted or when their environment becomes unpredictable. Repetitive behaviors may include repetitive movements, such as hand-flapping, or intense attachment to specific objects or activities, such as listening to music. These behaviors can interfere with learning and social participation.
- **Level 3:** Individuals at Level 3 often engage in highly repetitive and restrictive behaviors that dominate their daily lives. They may exhibit extreme distress when their routines are altered. Self-injurious behaviors, such as head-banging or biting, may also occur, particularly when they are unable to communicate discomfort or needs effectively. Unfamiliar environments can provoke extreme

distress, requiring constant supervision to manage safety.

4. Sensory Processing Challenges

Sensory sensitivities can have a profound impact on the daily lives of individuals with autism.

- **Level 1:** Individuals may be hypersensitive to specific sensory inputs, such as loud noises, bright lights, or certain textures. (Baranek et al., 2006) They may avoid certain environments (e.g., crowded places) due to sensory overload. Alternatively, they may also be hyposensitive and seek sensory input, such as by touching different textures or making loud noises. Think of it this way, hyper is too much and hypo is too little. Hypersensitivity tends to lead to avoidance while hyposensitivity will lead to someone seeking out the sensory input they need.
- **Level 2:** Sensory processing challenges can be more pronounced, with individuals experiencing significant discomfort from sensory stimuli that others may not notice. They may have difficulty filtering out background stimuli, making it challenging to focus inside busy environments. Sensory overload can lead to meltdowns or withdrawal from activities. Sensory overload is more frequent and visibly distressing, with individuals covering their ears, crying, screaming, or withdrawing from the stimuli. Withdrawal from an area can be described as bolting. Repetitive stimming behaviors, such as humming or tapping, are common ways to self-soothe.
- **Level 3:** Severe sensory aversions are common at this level. Individuals may become overwhelmed by even mild sensory input. They may rely on repetitive behaviors to self-soothe and regulate their sensory experiences. Managing sensory needs is crucial for maintaining their emotional and physical well-being. Controlled environments

and specialized sensory tools are critical for maintaining emotional stability and reducing distress in these individuals.

13

4

Chapter 4: Strategies to Overcome Challenges

Enhancing Communication
Developing effective communication skills is a key focus of interventions for individuals with autism.

For Level 1:

Encouraging the use of social stories or scripts can help individuals initiate and maintain conversations. Practicing social scripts for common interactions, such as greetings or small talk, can help build confidence. Practicing role-playing scenarios and using visual aids, such as charts or diagrams, can enhance comprehension of abstract concepts. Promoting self-expression through creative outlets, like writing or art, can also be helpful. Creative outlets like journaling or art can provide alternative ways of expression. Tools like visual organizers, planners, or visual apps can assist in clarifying thoughts and responses.

For Level 2:

Augmentative and alternative communication (AAC) tools, such as speech-generating devices or communication boards, can be used to support individuals with limited verbal skills. Visual supports such as Picture Exchange Communication Systems (PECS) can bridge communication gaps, while augmentative and alternative communication (AAC) devices give nonverbal individuals a voice. Simplified language, along with visual aids like picture schedules and social stories, can help individuals understand expectations and express themselves. Reinforcing communication attempts with positive feedback (verbal praise) ensures consistent progress.

For Level 3:

The focus of level 3 is often on developing basic communication skills to meet essential basic needs. This may include using gestures, symbols, signs, or Augmentative and Alternative Communication (AAC) devices to request items, express discomfort, or indicate preferences. Tools like speech-generating devices or communication boards allow individuals to select words, pictures, or symbols to express their needs, even without verbal language. The widespread availability of user-friendly, customizable AAC devices such as iPads equipped with Proloquo2Go or TouchChat has dramatically improved communication for individuals at Level 3. These devices provide individuals with a "voice" by enabling them to participate in decisions about their daily lives. This breakthrough has led to a marked reduction in frustration-driven behaviors and enhanced overall quality of life by empowering individuals to communicate their needs, preferences, and emotions effectively. Moreover, collaboration with speech-language pathologists can be instrumental in developing individualized communication interventions.

Building Social Skills

Developing social competence requires structured, supportive approaches tailored to the individual's abilities.

For Level 1:

Teaching perspective-taking and empathy can improve social interactions. Role-playing social scenarios and encouraging participation in structured group activities, such as clubs or classes, can provide opportunities to practice and reinforce social skills. Teaching emotional recognition, such as identifying facial expressions or tone of voice, enhances empathy and relationship-building. The development of structured social groups tailored to individuals with Level 1 autism, such as those offered by organizations like PEERS (Program for the Education and Enrichment of Relational Skills), has significantly enhanced quality of life. These programs teach practical social strategies and provide opportunities to practice them in real-world situations. Strategies such as this can lead to improved social confidence and meaningful relationships.

For Level 2:

Peer modeling, where typically developing peers demonstrate appropriate social behavior, can be an effective strategy. Social scripts to teach appropriate behaviors can be an effective social building tool by explaining expectations and outcomes while providing clarity and confidence. Breaking down complex social interactions into manageable steps and practicing them in safe, supportive environments can also be beneficial.

For Level 3:

The primary focus is on functional social interactions, which is the most basic level of a social interaction. For instance, acknowledging a hello. The goal is to prioritize simple interactions such as greeting others or making basic requests. Basic social behaviors like making eye contact or waving goodbye are emphasized through consistent practice in familiar environments. Doing this with trusted caregivers can help build comfort and competency in social settings because caregivers tend to be the foundation for building social trust. Sensory-friendly settings can help reduce anxiety during social interactions. If possible, sensory rooms can be developed to assist in these social interactions. Sensory rooms may consist of swings, wall pads with different textures, floor pads with different textures, wall lights, chalk boards, hands on interactive boards such as cranks, or various fidget toys.

Managing Behavioral Issues

Behavioral challenges can be addressed using a combination of proactive and reactive strategies.

For Level 1:

Positive reinforcement can be used to encourage flexibility and adaptability. Saying things like "good job being flexible" is a form of positive reinforcement. Gradual exposure to changes, with clear explanations and visual supports, can help individuals become more comfortable with new experiences. Reinforcing positive behaviors with rewards encourages cooperation. Teaching coping mechanisms, such as deep breathing or using fidget toys, can help manage frustration.

For Level 2:

Structured routines and visual schedules can provide a sense of predictability thus, reducing anxiety. For example, caregivers and educators can use visual supports, such as pictures or icons, to outline daily routines. They can also prepare individuals for changes with transition warnings by saying things like "In 10 minutes, we will switch activities". Identifying triggers for meltdowns and addressing them through environmental modifications or calming techniques can also help manage behaviors. Sensory integration techniques, such as deep pressure or weighted blankets, can help individuals self-regulate.

Behavior analysts can develop individualized plans to target specific behaviors. The integration of Applied Behavior Analysis (ABA) with visual aids has led to substantial improvements in adaptability. Over time, gradual exposure to small, managed changes in routine using visual schedules has reduced behavioral rigidity. This approach allows individuals to anticipate and prepare for transitions, fostering greater independence and reducing anxiety-driven behaviors.

For Level 3:

Behavior analysts can work with caregivers to create individualized behavior intervention plans (BIPs). These plans often include strategies for preventing problematic behaviors, teaching alternative behaviors, and managing crises. Addressing self-injurious behaviors requires identifying triggers and implementing preventative measures. Sensory-based strategies, like providing calming tactile objects, such as a soft brush or squishy ball, can reduce anxiety. Consistent reinforcement of replacement behaviors ensures progress. For example, reinforcing putting food items they no longer want back into their lunchbox verses dumping them on the floor.

Addressing Sensory Needs

Supporting sensory needs can significantly improve an individual's quality of life.

For Level 1:

Providing tools like noise-canceling headphones, fidget toys, sunglasses, or weighted blankets can help individuals manage sensory overload. These strategies end up becoming a coping mechanism to deal with discomfort. Creating sensory-friendly environments at home and at school can also promote comfort and focus by providing safe zones for self-regulation. Encouraging sensory-seeking behaviors in safe ways, such as using sensory bins or swings, supports emotional balance. Sensory bins may look like sandboxes or be filled with beans.

For Level 2:

Incorporating sensory breaks into daily routines allows individuals to self-regulate and maintain focus. This might look like having a music break, a video break, or a toy break. Fidget tools, textured items, or sensory bins can provide the input they need to stay engaged in tasks and activities. For example, a sensory bin might be different colored paperclips, this can help an individual who enjoys counting work on attention and focusing skills. Adapting environments, such as dimming lights or reducing noise with sound machines, works to minimize overstimulation. Tailored sensory diets designed by occupational therapists offer consistent input to help individuals stay regulated.

For Level 3:

Creating controlled sensory environments is essential for individuals at this level. Quiet rooms, dim lighting, and constant access to sensory tools, like compression clothing or chewable necklaces, help to ensure comfort and stability. Vocational bins may also be used. These bins can contain things like sorting activities, folding socks, counting clothes pins, or folding hand towels. Collaborating with occupational therapists can help identify specific sensory needs, allowing for effective design interventions. For instance, they might be able to tell you how to organize a sensory room that would be the most useful for a particular individual. You may also work with an occupational therapist to develop a sensory diet that can help meet an individual's sensory needs when it comes to food. A sensory diet can help assist the eating process in a more structured way. Minimizing sensory overload by creating calm, predictable environments is crucial for individuals at this level, as even minor sensory disruptions can lead to significant distress

5

Chapter 5: The Role of Caregivers, Educators, and Healthcare Professionals

Family Support Systems

Caregivers play a crucial role in fostering the development of individuals with autism. (Koegel et al., 2016) Caregivers are the backbone of support for these individuals. The emotional, social, and practical support they provide is foundational to an individual's success.

- **Building Routines:** Creating consistent routines and a safe home environment helps to provide structure and predictability, thereby reducing anxiety. Visual schedules, timers, and step-by-step instructions can make routines more manageable for individuals with autism.
- **Advocacy:** Caregivers are often the primary advocates for their loved ones by ensuring they receive appropriate support at school, in healthcare settings, and in the community. Understanding their rights and available resources is key to effective advocacy.
- **Training and Education:** Participating in and seeking out training programs, as well as other resources, helps caregivers learn effective

intervention techniques and strategies for managing challenges. Caregiver education also enhances their ability to respond to their loved one's unique needs and better support their child. Caregiver education is typically provided by a Board-Certified Behavior Analyst (BCBA) as part of their child's behavior intervention program (BIP).

Educational Strategies

Education is a critical component of support for individuals diagnosed with autism spectrum disorder. (Gray, 2010) Educators, such as behavior technicians, play an essential role in this process.

- **Individualized Education Plans (IEPs):** Developing and implementing IEPs helps to tailor the educational experience to each student's needs, strengths, and challenges. Goals within an IEP should be specific, measurable, and focused on improving academic, social, and adaptive skills.
- **Visual Supports and Differentiated Instruction:** Visual supports, such as charts, diagrams, and picture schedules, within the educational environment can enhance comprehension and engagement. Differentiated instruction, or flexible teaching methods, such as tailoring teaching methods to accommodate diverse learning styles, is also crucial for ensuring that students with autism can access the curriculum. Clear instructions can help these individuals stay focused on the tasks at hand.
- **Social Skills Training:** Educators can integrate social skills training into the school day by teaching social rules as well as encouraging peer interactions and inclusion. Educators can contrive opportunities for students to practice these skills in real-life situations or made-up scenarios to help foster understanding among peers. Social groups and activities are a good way to work on social skills. Programs and websites, such as Boom Learning, can teach social

skills as well as others that are required by the individual

Therapeutic Interventions

Healthcare professionals provide critical interventions that support communication, behavior, and overall development.

- **Speech Therapy:** Speech-language pathologists (SLPs) work to improve verbal and nonverbal communication skills. For individuals who are nonverbal, SLPs may introduce AAC devices to facilitate communication.
- **Occupational Therapy:** Occupational therapists focus on developing fine motor skills, improving sensory integration, and teaching daily living skills. They help individuals with autism become more independent by addressing both sensory and motor challenges.
- **Behavioral Therapy:** Applied Behavior Analysis (ABA) is a widely used behavioral intervention that focuses on improving specific behaviors, such as communication, social skills, and adaptive learning. ABA uses positive reinforcement to encourage desired behaviors and reduce problematic ones.

6

Chapter 6: An expanded exploration of Therapeutic Interventions

The Role of a Speech-Language Pathologist in Supporting Individuals with Autism

Speech-language pathologists (SLPs) play a critical role in the lives of individuals with autism spectrum disorder (ASD) by addressing communication challenges that impact daily life, social interactions, and personal development. Their work is highly individualized, catering to the unique strengths and needs of each person on the spectrum. SLPs support individuals with this disorder in multiple ways.

1. Assessment and Diagnosis

SLPs often conduct comprehensive evaluations to assess communication abilities. These assessments focus on:

- **Receptive Language:** The ability to understand spoken or written language, including following instructions or interpreting questions.
- **Expressive Language:** The ability to convey thoughts, needs, and

emotions using words, phrases, or gestures.

- **Nonverbal Communication:** Skills such as eye contact, facial expressions, and body language.
- **Social Communication (Pragmatics):** The use of language in social contexts, such as taking turns in conversation, understanding sarcasm, or adapting speech to different audiences.
- **Speech Clarity:** Assessing articulation, fluency, and intelligibility.

For nonverbal individuals, SLPs evaluate the potential for using augmentative and alternative communication (AAC) systems. These assessments help create a tailored intervention plan that aligns with the individual's developmental level and needs.

2. Developing Functional Communication

One of the primary goals for SLPs working with individuals with autism is fostering functional communication—the ability to express basic needs and preferences effectively. Strategies include:

- **Teaching Requests:** Helping individuals learn to ask for items or assistance, often starting with simple words, signs, or picture exchanges.
- **Expanding Vocabulary:** Gradually introducing new words or phrases to increase expressive capabilities.
- **AAC Devices:** Implementing and training individuals to use tools such as speech-generating devices, communication apps, or symbol-based systems like Picture Exchange Communication System (PECS).

Functional communication is particularly important for reducing frustration and challenging behaviors that arise when individuals cannot express themselves.

3. Enhancing Social Communication Skills

Social communication, or pragmatics, is a key area of difficulty for many individuals with autism. SLPs focus on:

- **Initiating and Maintaining Conversations:** Teaching these individuals how to start conversations, ask questions, and respond appropriately to others.
- **Turn-Taking and Sharing:** Practicing skills that promote reciprocity in social interactions.
- **Understanding Nonverbal Cues:** Helping individuals interpret facial expressions, gestures, and tone of voice.
- **Social Scripts:** Using pre-taught phrases or scenarios to navigate common social situations, such as ordering food at a restaurant or greeting someone.

For individuals with more advanced skills, SLPs might focus on understanding abstract social norms, such as recognizing sarcasm or adapting language for different audiences.

4. Addressing Speech and Language Development

SLPs help individuals with autism improve their verbal communication skills though interventions such as:

- **Articulation Therapy:** For individuals who can speak but struggle with clear pronunciation, SLPs work on improving speech clarity and enunciation.
- **Building Sentence Structure:** For those with limited language, SLPs help expand single words into meaningful sentences, usually starting with 3-word phrases and building from there.
- **Fluency Training:** Addressing speech disruptions, such as stuttering or hesitations, which can affect communication.

These therapies not only improve verbal communication but also build confidence in interacting with others.

5. Supporting Nonverbal Communication

For individuals who are nonverbal or have limited verbal skills, SLPs provide alternative methods of communication. This may include:

- **AAC Training:** Teaching individuals to use devices, apps, or communication boards effectively.
- **Sign Language:** Introducing simple signs to convey basic needs like bathroom, eat, or drink.
- **Gestures and Symbols:** Encouraging the use of pointing, head nodding, or picture-based systems to communicate.

Nonverbal communication interventions are essential for enabling individuals to participate in their environment and make choices about their daily lives.

6. Reducing Echolalia and Repetitive Language

Echolalia—repeating words or phrases—can be a common communication behavior in individuals with autism. SLPs work to:

- **Redirect Echolalia:** Transforming repeated phrases into functional communication. For example, teaching an individual to use repeated phrases like "I want that" appropriately.
- **Expand Beyond Repetition:** Encouraging spontaneous language by modeling new phrases and providing opportunities to practice.

This approach helps individuals develop more versatile and meaningful communication skills.

7. Collaboration with Families and Educators

SLPs are integral members of the care team, working closely with families, educators, and other professionals to ensure consistency in communication strategies. This collaboration includes:

- **Parent Training:** Teaching parents how to reinforce communication goals at home, such as using visual supports or modeling appropriate language.
- **Teacher Support:** Advising educators on classroom accommodations, such as seating arrangements, visual schedules, or AAC device integration.
- **Therapeutic Consistency:** Ensuring that strategies used in therapy sessions are applied consistently across all environments.

Effective collaboration maximizes the impact of speech therapy by creating a supportive network around the individual.

8. Long-Term Communication Goals

SLPs work to achieve long-term goals that align with the individual's developmental and life stages. Goals may include:

- **Independence:** Teaching communication strategies that enable individuals to express themselves without assistance.
- **Vocational Readiness:** Preparing individuals to use communication skills in the workplace, such as engaging with coworkers or understanding job-related instructions.
- **Self-Advocacy:** Empowering individuals to communicate their needs, preferences, and boundaries effectively.

Long-term progress often involves transitioning from therapy-focused sessions to applying communication skills in everyday life, otherwise known as generalization of the communication skills.

Case Example: A Holistic Role

Consider an 8-year-old child with Level 2 autism who struggles with both verbal and nonverbal communication. The SLP begins by introducing a PECS system to help the child request snacks or toys. Over time, the SLP expands the child's use of PECS to include expressing emotions, such as showing a picture of "happy" or "tired." Concurrently, the SLP works with the child's teacher to implement visual supports in the classroom, such as a daily schedule with pictures. At home, the SLP trains the parents to model simple sentences during play, like "Your turn" or "I want blocks." After six months, the child begins combining PECS symbols with verbal approximations, such as saying "want cookie" while pointing to the picture. This comprehensive approach enhances the child's ability to communicate across settings.

Speech-language pathologists are essential in helping individuals with autism navigate communication challenges, whether through verbal, nonverbal, or alternative methods. By tailoring interventions to each individual's needs and collaborating with families and educators, SLPs help create meaningful improvements in quality of life, social relationships, and independence.

The Role of an Occupational Therapist in Supporting Individuals with Autism

Occupational therapists (OTs) play a crucial role in helping individuals with autism spectrum disorder (ASD) develop the skills needed to navigate daily life. Their work focuses on enhancing independence, addressing sensory processing challenges, and improving social and functional abilities.

1. Addressing Sensory Processing Challenges

Many individuals with autism experience sensory processing difficulties, such as hypersensitivity or hyposensitivity to stimuli like sound, touch, light, or movement. OTs are trained to assess these sensory needs and create tailored interventions, often referred to as a "sensory diet." A sensory diet includes activities designed to help regulate an individual's sensory input, such as using weighted blankets, fidget tools, or deep-pressure techniques. These interventions aim to help individuals achieve a state of sensory regulation, which is essential for focus, learning, and participation in daily activities.

2. Enhancing Daily Living Skills

OTs work on developing the fine motor, gross motor, and adaptive skills required for everyday activities. These include self-care tasks, such as dressing, eating, brushing teeth, and using the bathroom (activities of daily living - ADL's). For example, an OT might teach a child with autism how to button a shirt using hand-over-hand guidance before gradually reducing assistance. The focus is on breaking tasks into smaller, manageable steps and practicing them consistently to build independence.

3. Improving Social and Play Skills

Play is an essential part of childhood development, and for many children with autism, structured play interventions guided by an OT can foster social skills, creativity, and engagement. For example, an OT might facilitate turn-taking activities, cooperative games, or pretend play to encourage interaction with peers. These sessions often include sensory-friendly toys or activities that match the child's interests to maintain motivation and comfort.

4. Addressing Fine and Gross Motor Skills

Many individuals with autism struggle with motor coordination and strength. OTs provide exercises and activities to improve these skills. This is crucial for tasks such as handwriting, using utensils, or climbing playground equipment. For instance, activities like threading beads or using therapy putty help refine fine motor skills and build hand strength. Obstacle courses or balance exercises improve gross motor coordination.

5. Supporting School and Academic Participation

OTs collaborate with teachers and special education staff to create strategies that enable students with autism to succeed in the classroom. This may involve adapting the environment (providing noise-canceling headphones to reduce distractions), modifying activities (using larger pencils or grip assists for better grip), or teaching self-regulation techniques (using a sensory break schedule). These accommodations ensure that students can engage in learning despite sensory or motor challenges.

6. Promoting Emotional Regulation

OTs are skilled at helping individuals with autism manage their emotions and behaviors. This is often achieved through sensory integration therapy, which helps individuals process sensory input in a way that is less overwhelming. OTs might teach calming techniques, such as deep breathing or using a sensory tool such as a squishy toy to help individuals regulate emotions and prevent meltdowns.

7. Collaboration with Families and Other Professionals

Collaboration is a cornerstone of occupational therapy. OTs work closely with families to ensure that therapeutic strategies are practiced consistently at home. They also partner with other professionals, such as speech-language pathologists, educators, and behavioral therapists, to create a comprehensive intervention plan. By integrating efforts, OTs help ensure that individuals with this disorder receive consistent support across all environments.

Occupational therapists play an indispensable role in helping individuals with autism develop the skills necessary to navigate their world. By addressing sensory needs, enhancing daily living and motor skills, and promoting emotional regulation, OTs enable individuals with autism to achieve greater independence and participation in their communities. Their holistic and collaborative approach ensures that individuals with autism and their families are supported in meaningful and practical ways.

The Role of Behavior Technicians and Board-Certified Behavior Analysts (BCBAs) in Supporting Individuals with Autism

Behavior technicians and Board-Certified Behavior Analysts (BCBAs) are integral members of the care team for individuals with autism spectrum disorder (ASD). Both roles focus on implementing and managing Applied Behavior Analysis (ABA), a widely recognized evidence-based intervention practice for those with autism. Below is a more in-depth explanation of their responsibilities, contributions, and collaborative efforts in improving the quality of life for individuals with autism.

Behavior Technicians: Frontline Implementation
Responsibilities and Contributions:

Behavior technicians, often referred to as Registered Behavior Technicians (RBTs), work directly with individuals with autism to implement ABA programs designed by a BCBA. Their responsibilities include:

1. Delivering Direct Intervention:

- Behavior technicians work with individuals in one-on-one or small group settings, teaching functional communication, social skills, and daily living skills. For example, they might help a child learn to request a preferred item using verbal cues or a Picture Exchange Communication System (PECS).

- They use positive reinforcement strategies to encourage desired behaviors and reduce maladaptive ones, such as aggression or self-injury.

2. Data Collection:

- A critical part of the RBT's role is collecting accurate, detailed data on the individual's progress. This includes tracking the frequency, duration, or intensity of specific behaviors to evaluate the effectiveness of interventions.

3. Promoting Generalization:

- RBTs help individuals apply learned skills across different settings, such as at home, school, or in the community. For instance, teaching a child to greet peers during playdates as well as in the classroom ensures that skills are transferable and meaningful.

4. Implementing Behavior Reduction Plans:

- When challenging behaviors occur, RBTs follow behavior intervention plans (BIPs) developed by the BCBA. These plans include proactive and reactive strategies tailored to each individual's needs, such as redirecting a tantrum to a more appropriate form of communication.

Impact on Individuals with Autism:

Behavior technicians serve as the primary point of contact for individuals with autism during intervention sessions. Their consistent presence and rapport-building efforts help create a trusting environment where individuals feel supported and motivated to learn.

Board Certified Behavior Analysts (BCBAs): Supervisors and Designers of Intervention Plans

Responsibilities and Contributions:

BCBAs are highly trained professionals responsible for designing, monitoring, and supervising ABA programs. Their responsibilities include:

1. Conducting Functional Behavior Assessments (FBA):

- BCBAs analyze the causes and functions of specific behaviors. For example, if a child frequently engages in tantrums, the BCBA evaluates whether the behavior is triggered by sensory overload, escape from tasks, or the need for attention. This assessment informs the creation of targeted interventions.

2. Developing Individualized Treatment Plans:

- BCBAs design comprehensive ABA programs tailored to the individual's unique needs. These plans include measurable goals, such as improving communication, reducing self-injurious behavior, or enhancing social skills. For instance, a BCBA might develop a plan to teach a nonverbal child to use an AAC device to request snacks or toys.

3. Supervising Behavior Technicians:

- BCBAs provide ongoing supervision to RBTs, ensuring interventions are implemented correctly and ethically. This includes regular team meetings, direct observation of sessions, and feedback to enhance effectiveness.

4. Analyzing Data and Adjusting Programs:

- Using data collected by RBTs, BCBAs evaluate progress toward goals and make necessary adjustments. For example, if a skill is not being mastered, the BCBA might modify the teaching approach or reinforcement schedule.

5. Training Caregivers and Educators:

- BCBAs provide training to parents, teachers, and other caregivers, empowering them to reinforce intervention strategies in everyday interactions. This might involve teaching a parent how to manage meltdowns or helping a teacher adapt classroom tasks to an individual's needs.

Impact on Individuals with Autism:

The expertise of a BCBA ensures that interventions are both effective and evidence based. Their role is essential for creating individualized programs that address core challenges in communication, behavior, and social interaction while promoting long-term success.

Collaboration Between BCBAs and Behavior Technicians

The collaboration between BCBAs and RBTs ensures a seamless and effective approach to intervention. BCBAs provide the strategic oversight and clinical direction, while RBTs carry out the daily implementation. This dynamic relationship allows for:

- **Consistency in Intervention:** RBTs deliver interventions consistently under the guidance of the BCBA.
- **Efficient Problem-Solving:** BCBAs analyze data collected by RBTs to make real-time adjustments, ensuring progress toward goals.
- **Comprehensive Support:** Together, they address the full spectrum of needs, from behavior management to skill acquisition.

Case Example: Practical Application

Consider an 8-year-old boy with Level 2 autism who struggles with aggression during transitions. The BCBA conducts an FBA and identifies that the aggression occurs when he is asked to stop a preferred activity. The BCBA designs an intervention plan that includes:

- **Teaching a Replacement Behavior:** Using an AAC device or verbal language to request more time instead of exhibiting aggression.
- **Reinforcing Positive Behavior:** RBTs provide praise or access to a reward when the child uses the AAC device appropriately.
- **Gradual Desensitization:** RBTs work with the child to gradually increase tolerance for transitions, pairing them with preferred activities.

Over time, the child learns to request more time using the AAC device, reducing instances of aggression and making transitions smoother.

7

Chapter 7: Building Inclusive Communities

Promoting Awareness and Acceptance
Creating a more inclusive society for individuals with autism requires a multi-faceted approach that combines awareness, acceptance, and actionable change. Inclusivity begins with understanding. We must educate communities about autism and break down stereotypes surrounding the disorder. Promoting awareness of autism helps dispel myths, combat stereotypes, reduce stigma, and create a supportive environment for individuals on the spectrum. It Involves recognizing the unique contributions of individuals with the disorder.

- **Educational Campaigns:** Schools, workplaces, and community organizations can organize educational campaigns or workshops to raise awareness about autism. Providing accurate information and challenging stereotypes can help foster a culture of acceptance. Peer education in schools encourages neurotypical students to understand and embrace differences. Thus, fostering friendships and reducing bullying. Similarly, workplaces can adopt neurodiversity initiatives that celebrate the strengths of employees with autism, such as their attention to detail or problem-solving skills.

- **Autism Acceptance Events:** Community events such as World Autism Awareness Day and Autism Acceptance Month are opportunities to celebrate neurodiversity and promote the inclusion of individuals with autism. Communities can hold events that highlight the strengths and talents of individuals on the spectrum such as autism-friendly art exhibitions, talent shows, and career fairs. These events create platforms for individuals with autism to showcase their talents and engage with the broader community.

Creating Autism-Friendly Environments

Inclusive environments are those that accommodate the sensory, social, and behavioral needs of individuals with autism.

- **Sensory-Friendly Spaces:** Sensory-friendly adaptations can make public spaces more accessible. Designing quiet spaces in schools, libraries, workplaces, and public areas such as parks, can provide individuals with a place to retreat when feeling overwhelmed. Sensory-friendly movie screenings, playgrounds, and events are also becoming more common which helps ensure that individuals with autism can participate in community activities. Museums, theaters, and shopping malls can designate quiet hours or create sensory rooms to accommodate individuals with heightened sensitivities. Restaurants and airports can offer sensory kits or designated calming areas. There are currently restaurants that advertise themselves as "Autism Welcoming" through the Autism Alliance and AutismWelcoming.org. One such restaurant is California Pizza Kitchen at the Natick Mall in Massachusetts. Schools and community centers can design playgrounds that include sensory-friendly equipment, such as swings or textured pathways. Additionally, public transportation systems can train staff to better assist individuals with autism, ensuring they feel safe and supported while traveling.

- **Training Staff in Autism-Friendly Practices:** Staff at schools, healthcare facilities, and community centers should receive training on autism-friendly practices, including how to communicate effectively, provide appropriate support, and manage challenging behaviors. This training ensures that individuals with autism receive consistent support across different settings. One such training is called "Safety Care".

- **Employment Inclusion:** Employment inclusion is another critical component of building inclusive communities. Programs like Project SEARCH and Autism at Work, initiatives by companies such as Microsoft and SAP, have demonstrated the potential of individuals with autism in the workforce. These programs provide job training, mentorship, and tailored support to help individuals succeed in various industries. Small businesses and local organizations can also play a role by hiring individuals with autism along with creating structured, supportive work environments. Supported employment services, such as job coaching or on-the-job assistance, further enhance the likelihood of success.

Inclusive communities prioritize the voices and perspectives of individuals with autism. Advocacy groups often include individuals with autism in leadership roles, ensuring their experiences shape policies and initiatives. Public forums and decision-making bodies can create opportunities for individuals on the spectrum to share their insights on accessibility, education, and employment. By actively involving individuals with autism in shaping their communities, society moves closer to genuine inclusivity. Through education, adaptation, and collaboration, communities can create environments where individuals with autism feel valued, understood, and empowered to reach their full potential.

8

Chapter 8: Resources for Individuals with Autism at Every Level

Navigating the available resources for individuals with autism can be overwhelming for families, caregivers, and individuals themselves. These resources range from therapeutic services to educational programs and community support systems. Tailoring resources to the needs of individuals at different levels of autism ensures that they receive the appropriate care and support necessary for their growth and well-being.

1. Early Intervention Programs

Early intervention is crucial for children diagnosed with this disorder. These programs focus on addressing developmental delays and challenges in communication, social interaction, and behavior.

Examples of Early Intervention Resources:

- **Applied Behavior Analysis (ABA):** A widely used therapy that focuses on improving specific behaviors and skills through positive reinforcement.

- **Early Start Denver Model (ESDM)**: A play-based intervention designed for children aged 12-48 months.
- **State-Funded Early Intervention Programs**: Available under the Individuals with Disabilities Education Act (IDEA) in the United States, these services often include speech therapy, occupational therapy, and behavioral interventions.

How to Access: Families can consult pediatricians, developmental specialists, or local health departments to connect with early intervention services.

2. Educational Resources

Education plays a vital role in helping individuals with autism achieve their full potential. Educational resources vary depending on the individual's level of need. Early intervention programs, such as ABA and ESDM, are critical for improving outcomes in young children with autism (Smith & Iadarola, 2015).

For Level 1:

- **Inclusive Classrooms:** Schools provide accommodations, such as Individualized Education Plans (IEPs), to support learning alongside neurotypical peers.
- **Assistive Technology:** Tools like apps for communication, social skills training, and time management.
- **Specialized Curriculum**: Programs like Social Thinking are used to enhance social awareness and relationship-building skills.

For Level 2:

- **Specialized Classrooms:** Smaller class sizes and individualized teaching approaches cater to their needs.

- **Visual Supports**: Tools like visual schedules and Picture Exchange Communication Systems (PECS) to aid understanding and communication.
- **Applied Behavior Analysis (ABA):** Offered within educational settings to address behavior and learning challenges.

For Level 3:

- **Specialized Schools:** Institutions tailored to nonverbal individuals and those requiring substantial support. In Massachusetts, one such school is the Nashoba Learning Group or NLG.
- **One-on-One Instruction:** Intensive teaching to focus on life skills and functional communication.
- **Assistive Technology:** Speech-generating devices and other tools to facilitate communication and learning.

3. Therapeutic Resources

Therapeutic services address the core challenges of autism, such as communication difficulties, sensory sensitivities, and repetitive behaviors.

Speech and Language Therapy:

- Focuses on improving verbal and nonverbal communication skills.
- Includes augmentative and alternative communication (AAC) for nonverbal individuals.

Occupational Therapy (OT):

- Enhances fine motor skills, daily living activities, and sensory processing abilities.
- Incorporates sensory integration techniques to manage sensitivities.

Behavioral Therapy:

- Applied Behavior Analysis (ABA) is the gold standard for addressing behavior-related challenges.
- Cognitive Behavioral Therapy (CBT) is effective for individuals with Level 1 autism to manage anxiety and emotional regulation.

4. Support Groups and Community Resources

Connecting with others in the autism community can provide emotional support, practical advice, and a sense of belonging.

For Families and Caregivers:

- Local and national organizations, such as Autism Speaks and the Autism Society, offer resources and support groups.
- Parent training programs help families understand and address the unique needs of their loved ones.

For Individuals with Autism:

- Peer support groups provide a space to share experiences and build connections.
- Community centers and recreational programs offer tailored activities for individuals at all levels.

5. Employment and Vocational Resources

Employment programs help individuals with autism, particularly adolescents and adults, gain skills and access meaningful job opportunities.

For Level 1:

- Vocational training programs like Project SEARCH prepare individuals for competitive employment.
- Autism-friendly employers, such as companies with neurodiversity hiring initiatives.

For Level 2:

- Supported employment services with job coaches to provide on-the-job assistance.
- Transition programs that teach job-related skills as part of high school IEPs.

For Level 3:

- Sheltered workshops offering structured environments for work tasks.
- Day programs focusing on skill-building and supervised employment.

6. Financial and Legal Resources

Managing the financial and legal aspects of care is critical for families of individuals with autism.

Financial Assistance:

- Supplemental Security Income (SSI): Provides monthly payments for individuals with disabilities.
- Medicaid Waivers: Fund services such as therapy, respite care, and assistive devices.

Legal Advocacy:

- Organizations like Disability Rights groups offer guidance on accessing education, healthcare, and housing rights.
- Guardianship and special needs trusts help families plan for long-term care and financial stability.

7. Assistive Technology

Technology can empower individuals with autism by enhancing communication, independence, and learning.

For Level 1:

- Apps for time management, social skills, and emotional regulation.
- Online learning platforms tailored to individual learning styles.

For Level 2 and Level 3:

- Speech-generating devices and AAC tools for nonverbal individuals.
- Sensory aids such as weighted blankets, noise-canceling headphones, and tactile toys.

8. Healthcare Resources

Access to specialized healthcare services is vital for addressing co-occurring conditions and promoting overall well-being.

- **Developmental Pediatricians:** Experts in diagnosing and treating autism-related issues.
- **Autism-Friendly Clinics:** Healthcare providers trained to accommodate sensory and communication needs.
- **Mental Health Services:** Therapists and psychiatrists specializing in autism to manage co-conditions like anxiety or depression.

9. How to Find Resources

Finding the right resources requires persistence and networking. Here are steps to guide families and individuals:

1. **Contact Local Organizations**: Many nonprofits and advocacy groups maintain directories of services.
2. **Speak with Professionals:** Pediatricians, therapists, and educators can recommend resources tailored to specific needs.
3. **Leverage Online Tools:** Websites like Autism Speaks, Understood.org, and government portals provide comprehensive information.
4. **Network with Other Families:** Joining support groups can help families learn from others' experiences and discover additional resources.

This chapter highlights the diverse range of resources available to individuals with autism and their families. Leveraging these resources can enhance quality of life, promote independence, and ensure access to opportunities for individuals at every level of the spectrum.

9

Conclusion

Autism Spectrum Disorder is a multifaceted condition that affects each individual differently. Understanding the levels of autism and the challenges they face is the first step toward providing meaningful support. By implementing tailored strategies and fostering inclusive communities, we can empower individuals with autism to lead fulfilling lives. Every individual on the autism spectrum has unique strengths and contributions to offer. It is our responsibility as a society to ensure that they have the support they need to thrive. A collective effort from caregivers, educators, healthcare professionals, and society at large is essential to create a world where individuals with autism are valued and supported for who they are.

I hope you found this book informative and helpful. If so, please leave a favorable review for the book on Amazon. I would be very grateful and appreciative if you did!

References

American Psychiatric Association. (2013). *Diagnostic and statistical manual of mental disorders* (5th ed.). Arlington, VA: American Psychiatric Publishing.

- Provides the diagnostic criteria for autism spectrum disorder, including the classification of levels.

American Speech-Language-Hearing Association. (n.d.). *Autism.* Retrieved from https://www.asha.org/Practice-Portal/Clinical-Topics/Autism/

- A comprehensive resource on the role of SLPs in autism, covering assessment, intervention, and use of AAC.

American Speech-Language-Hearing Association. (n.d.). *Augmentative and alternative communication (AAC).* Retrieved from https://www.asha.org/Practice-Portal/Clinical-Topics/Augmentative-and-Alternative-Communication/

- Details AAC systems and strategies for individuals with communication challenges, including autism.

Autism Speaks. (n.d.). *Applied behavior analysis (ABA): Overview and benefits.* Retrieved from https://www.autismspeaks.org

- An accessible resource for families to understand the basics of ABA therapy and its role in supporting individuals with autism.

Baranek, G. T., David, F. J., Poe, M. D., Stone, W. L., & Watson, L. R. (2006). Sensory experiences questionnaire: Discriminating sensory features in young children with autism, developmental delays, and typical development. *Journal of Child Psychology and Psychiatry, 47*(6), 591–601. https://doi.org/10.1111/j.1469-7610.2005.01546.x

- Discusses sensory processing issues in autism and provides evidence for the prevalence of these challenges.

Behavior Analyst Certification Board. (2023). *BCBA task list (5th edition).* Retrieved from https://www.bacb.com

- Outlines the responsibilities and competencies required of BCBAs.

Bondy, A., & Frost, L. (2001). The picture exchange communication system. *Behavior Modification, 25*(5), 725-744. https://doi.org/10.1177/0145445501255004

- Discusses the development and implementation of PECS for individuals with autism.

Carr, J. E., & Nosik, M. R. (2017). Professional credentialing of practicing behavior analysts. *Policy Insights from the Behavioral and Brain Sciences, 4*(1), 3-8. https://doi.org/10.1177/2372732216683342

- Discusses the role and importance of professional certification in ABA practices.

Case-Smith, J., & Arbesman, M. (2008). Evidence-based review of interventions for autism used in or of relevance to occupational therapy. *American Journal of Occupational Therapy, 62*(4), 416-429. https://doi.org/10.5014/ajot.62.4.416

- a comprehensive review that examines evidence-based interventions for autism relevant to occupational therapy, highlighting strategies that address sensory, motor, and social challenges to improve daily functioning and quality of life.

Centers for Disease Control and Prevention. (2020). *Autism spectrum disorder (ASD): Data and statistics.* Retrieved from https://www.cdc.gov/ncbddd/autism/data.html

- Offers statistical insights into the prevalence of autism and its demographic variations.

Cooper, J. O., Heron, T. E., & Heward, W. L. (2020). *Applied behavior analysis* (3rd ed.). Pearson.

- A foundational textbook that explains the principles and practices of ABA, including the roles of BCBAs and behavior technicians.

Dawson, G., & Bernier, R. (2013). Development of social brain circuitry in autism. *Trends in Neurosciences, 36*(4), 211–219. https://doi.org/10.1016/j.tins.2012.12.005

- Explores the neurological underpinnings of social challenges in autism, providing insight into brain development.

Gray, C. (2010). *The new social story book.* Arlington, TX: Future Horizons.

- A practical resource for using social stories to teach social skills to individuals with autism.

Koegel, L. K., Matos-Fredeen, R., Lang, R., & Koegel, R. L. (2016). Interventions for children with autism spectrum disorders in inclusive school settings. *Cognitive and Behavioral Practice, 19*(3), 401-412. https://doi.org/10.1016/j.cbpra.2010.10.003

- Examines effective interventions for supporting children with autism in inclusive educational environments.

Leaf, J. B., Leaf, R., McEachin, J., Taubman, M., & Ala'i-Rosales, S. (2018). ABA is a science and, therefore, progressive. *Journal of Autism and Developmental Disorders, 48*(12), 4230-4237. https://doi.org/10.1007/s10803-018-3683-5

- Explores advancements in ABA practices for individuals with autism.

Light, J., & McNaughton, D. (2014). Communicative competence for individuals who require augmentative and alternative communication: A new definition for a new era of communication? *Augmentative and Alternative Communication, 30*(1), 1-18. https://doi.org/10.3109/07434618.2014.885080

- Examines AAC tools and their role in enhancing communication skills.

Lord, C., Elsabbagh, M., Baird, G., & Veenstra-Vanderweele, J. (2018). Autism spectrum disorder. *The Lancet, 392*(10146), 508-520. https://doi.org/10.1016/S0140-6736(18)31129-2

- Provides a comprehensive overview of autism, including its diagnosis, causes, and interventions.

National Autism Center. (2015). *National standards project, phase 2: Addressing the need for evidence-based practice guidelines for autism spectrum disorder.* Randolph, MA: National Autism Center.

- Details evidence-based interventions and their effectiveness in treating autism.

Paul, R., & Norbury, C. F. (2012). *Language disorders from infancy through adolescence: Listening, speaking, reading, writing, and communicating* (4th ed.). St. Louis, MO: Elsevier.

- Includes chapters on pragmatic language development and interventions for individuals with autism.

Rogers, S. J., & Dawson, G. (2010). *Early start Denver model for young children with autism: Promoting language, learning, and engagement.* New York, NY: Guilford Press.

- Outlines the Early Start Denver Model, an intervention for young children with autism.

Schaaf, R. C., & Miller, L. J. (2005). Occupational therapy using a sensory integrative approach for children with developmental disabilities. *Mental Retardation and Developmental Disabilities Research Reviews, 11*(2), 143-148. https://doi.org/10.1002/mrdd.20067

- a study that explores the use of sensory integration approaches in occupational therapy to support children with developmental disabilities, including autism, focusing on improving sensory processing to enhance their functional and adaptive skills.

Smith, T., & Iadarola, S. (2015). Evidence base update for autism spectrum disorder. *Journal of Clinical Child & Adolescent Psychology, 44*(6), 897–922. https://doi.org/10.1080/15374416.2015.1077448

- Reviews the evidence base for various autism treatments, including behavioral and educational interventions.

Sundberg, M. L. (2008). *VB-MAPP: Verbal behavior milestones assessment and placement program.* AVB Press.

- Describes a widely used assessment tool in ABA that helps BCBAs design individualized intervention plans.

Understood.org. (n.d.). *Sensory processing issues explained.* Retrieved from https://www.understood.org

- An excellent resource for understanding sensory processing challenges and strategies for support.

Vollmer, T. R., & Smith, R. G. (1996). Some current themes in functional analysis research. *Research in Developmental Disabilities, 17*(3), 177–192. https://doi.org/10.1016/0891-4222(95)00044-5

- Discusses the use of functional behavior assessments in understanding and addressing challenging behaviors.

Volkmar, F. R., Paul, R., Rogers, S. J., & Pelphrey, K. A. (Eds.). (2014). *Handbook of autism and pervasive developmental disorders* (4th ed.).

Hoboken, NJ: Wiley.

* A comprehensive reference on autism, covering a wide range of topics from diagnosis to intervention strategies.

World Health Organization. (2021). *Autism spectrum disorders fact sheet.* Retrieved from https://www.who.int/news-room/fact-sheets/detail/autism-spectrum-disorders

* Provides an international perspective on autism, including prevalence, causes, and public health approaches.

Zwaigenbaum, L., Bauman, M. L., Stone, W. L., Yirmiya, N., Estes, A., Hansen, R. L., ... & Wetherby, A. (2015). Early identification of autism spectrum disorder: Recommendations for practice and research. *Pediatrics, 136*(S1), S10-S40. https://doi.org/10.1542/peds.2014-3667C

* Discusses the importance of early identification and intervention for improving outcomes in autism.

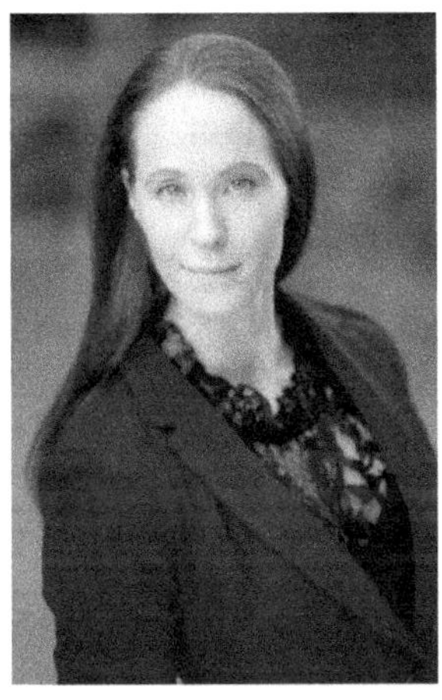

About the Author

Hello and welcome to my very first book. My name is Andrea Abella Marie. I am so excited that you decided to invest in this subject matter. It is a topic that I hold close to my heart considering I have several family members diagnosed with Autism Spectrum Disorder (ASD). I was inspired to write this book because of them.

I have been working as a behavior technician/case manager since January of 2022. I started working in the field after attending an Applied Behavior Analysis course while completing my Master's Degree in Public Health. I took my 40 hour Registered Behavior Technician course through the Autism Partnership Foundation in May of 2022.

I mostly work with nonverbal adults (Level 3) ages 22 and above in a clinic setting. Over the years, I have seen a variety of behaviors, helped implement behavior intervention plans (BIP's), been a job coach, and assisted my clients in their volunteer work. Integrating my clients into the community is just one vision of my workplace.

www.ingramcontent.com/pod-product-compliance
Lightning Source LLC
Chambersburg PA
CBHW051659250726
48653CB00007B/2743